Diabetic-Friendly Diet Guide for Adults

Empowering Your Health A Nutrient-Rich Guide to Managing Diabetes in Adulthood

Mila Moore

Table of Contents

Introduction

Chapter 1.Understanding Diabctes and
Diet
Importance of a Balanced Diet

Chapter 2. The Basics of Diabetes
Nutrition
Carbohydrates, Proteins, and Fats: Finding
the Right Balance
Glycemic Index and Glycemic Load
Explained

Chapter 3. Building a Healthy Plate
Portion Control and Plate Method
Incorporating a Variety of Foods

Chapter 4. Smart Food Choices

Best Carbohydrate Sources for Stable Blood Sugar

Lean Proteins for Sustained Energy

Heart-Healthy Fats

Chapter 5. Meal Planning and Preparation

Weekly Meal Planning Tips

Quick and Easy Diabetic-Friendly Recipes

Chapter 6. Snacking Strategies

Smart Snack Options for Between Meals

Managing Cravings and Emotional Eating

Chapter 7. Recipes for Success

Breakfast Ideas

Lunch and Dinner Recipes

Snack and Dessert Options

Conclusion

Taking Charge of Your Diabetes Journey

INTRODUCTION

Hello, and welcome to "Nourishing Vitality: Your Comprehensive Guide to a Diabetic-Friendly Diet." Our most valuable asset in the complex fabric of life is our state of health. In terms of health, overcoming diabetes management challenges and embracing well-being with open arms are both possible outcomes.

You'll set out on a transforming journey inside the pages of this book—one that goes beyond simple dietary recommendations to become a profound knowledge of how nutrition affects your journey toward managing your diabetes. In this section, we explore freedom from limitations and the power of empowerment, where information serves as your best ally.

You have an unyielding energy and a resolve that drives your search for a better future as adults negotiating the complexities of living with diabetes. This manual was created with you in mind. Every chapter and phrase in the book of your mind is a lighthouse of wisdom pointing the way to improved overall vitality, prolonged energy, and blood sugar control.

Together, we'll investigate the artistry of preparing meals that uplift the soul as well as the body. We'll explore the science behind mindful eating, portion control, and wise food choices, as well as the effects of physical activity, hydration, and mental health on your road to managing your diabetes.

You'll navigate the maze of nutritional options with newfound assurance if you are armed with medical specialists' insights, doable techniques, and delectable dishes customized to your requirements. You'll be equipped with the knowledge necessary to make decisions that are in line with your health, whether you're perusing a restaurant menu, seeking refuge in your kitchen, or navigating the difficulties of social situations.

This manual is a road map for recovering your sense of control over your health, not merely a collection of facts. In order to manage diabetes with grace and resiliency, let's set out on this adventure together, arming ourselves with information, enjoying the beauty of balanced eating, and appreciating life's flavors.

CHAPTER ONE

The significance of a balanced diet is discussed in Chapter 1: Understanding Diabetes and Diet.

Few diseases have as much relevance in the complex dance of health and wellness as diabetes. Diabetes, which affects millions of people worldwide, demands not just attention but also a thorough comprehension of its complexities. We lay the groundwork for understanding the symbiotic link between diabetes and food as we begin this informative trip through the first chapter.

Understanding Diabetes: Uncovering Its Complexities

A feature of diabetes, both type 1 and type 2, is fluctuating blood sugar levels. Insulin deficiency causes type 1 diabetes, which is brought on by an immune system attack on cells that make insulin. Insulin resistance, in which the body's cells do not respond to insulin as well as they should, frequently leads to type 2 diabetes.

This chapter clarifies the mechanisms at work so you may understand the physiology of diabetes from the ground up.

Diet: A Wellness Catalyst

According to the proverb, "We are what we eat." This statement has deep meaning when seen in the context of diabetes. A balanced diet is a tactical instrument for controlling blood sugar levels and advancing general health, not just a lifestyle choice. Every bite you take has the potential to affect your health, so choosing what you eat is crucial to achieving stability and energy.

What Is a Balanced Diet's Function?

Imagine a skillfully performed orchestra where each instrument contributes to a melodic harmony. Similar to this, a balanced diet arranges nutrients in perfect harmony to ensure that your body's processes run smoothly. Considering diabetes, a balanced diet attempts to avoid energy slumps, regulate blood sugar increases, and promote organ health. Your allies will be nutrient-rich foods since they manage your blood sugar levels and provide you with long-lasting energy.

The Dance of Proteins, Carbohydrates, and Fats

The fundamental components of your food are carbohydrates, proteins, and lipids, each of which has a specific function. Blood sugar levels are directly influenced by carbohydrates; proteins help repair and maintain muscles; and fats help the body absorb nutrients. When you master the balance of these macronutrients, you have the ability to create meals that support stable blood sugar levels and general wellbeing.

Beyond Blood Sugar: Whole-Body Advantages

A balanced diet is a catalyst for overall well being rather than just a way to keep blood sugar levels stable. The advantages of a balanced diet are revealed in this chapter. from strengthening brain and immunological resilience to enhancing cardiovascular health. Adopting a nutritious diet opens up a world of benefits that permeate all aspects of your life.

You'll leave this chapter with not just a grasp of diabetes and nutrition but also a fresh respect for the enormous influence your food choices have. With the right information, you're ready to set out on a path to a balanced and empowered lifestyle, where each mouthful becomes a chance to promote your wellbeing.

CHAPTER TWO

The basics of diabetes nutrition are discussed in Chapter 2, along with finding the right balance of carbohydrates, proteins, and fats and an explanation of the glycemic index and glycemic load.

Understanding how carbs, proteins, and fats interact is like possessing the key to a beautiful symphony in the complex mosaic of managing diabetes. The delicate balance of these macronutrients is revealed in Chapter 2, along with insights into the intricacies of glycemic index and glycemic load. This chapter goes deeply into the foundation of diabetic nutrition.

The Blood Sugar Conductor: Carbohydrates

Your body's main energy source, carbohydrates, has a significant impact on how much sugar is in your blood. Your connection with carbohydrates is crucial if you are controlling diabetes. This chapter guides you through the whole range of carbohydrates, from simple sugars to complex carbs. FBERs—helping you make decisions that maintain prolonged energy levels and stable blood sugar levels

Building Blocks of Vitality: Proteins

Proteins, the builders of your body's structural foundation, have a special place in a diabetic diet. In addition to helping maintain muscular strength, proteins aid in satiety and can control blood sugar levels. The delicate relationship between proteins and diabetes is revealed in this chapter, enabling you to incorporate these necessary nutrients into your meals to improve your general wellbeing.

Unveiling the Healthy Aspect of "Fats"

Although sometimes misunderstood, fats are a crucial component of a diabetic diet. Beyond being high in calories, certain fats promote heart health and help the body absorb fat-soluble vitamins. This chapter guides you through the maze of fats and directs you to sources that fuel you while keeping blood sugar levels in check.

Impact of Glycemic Index (GI): Decoding

Your decisions about carbohydrates are guided by the glycemic index. It measures how rapidly a meal containing carbohydrates increases blood sugar levels. This chapter explores the idea of GI, assisting you in identifying high-GI and low-GI meals so you may make informed choices that will stabilize blood sugar and encourage prolonged energy.

Glycemic load (GL): A comprehensive view

While GI offers useful information, Glycemic Load considers portion sizes and offers a more thorough knowledge of a food's effect on blood sugar. This chapter debunks GL, enabling you to think about both the type and amount of carbs ingested and providing a more complex view of the diabetic diet.

construction of a Harmonious Plate

You'll learn how to create a harmonious plate as you go through this chapter. It becomes second nature to balance proteins, lipids, and carbs while taking GI and GL factors into account. You'll leave with the knowledge necessary to choose meals that feed your body, support stable blood sugar levels, and encourage the joy of eating with intention.

You get closer to understanding the complex dance of a diabetic diet with every page you read. You get a comprehensive understanding of how to fuel your body while gently managing your diabetic journey as you weave together the threads of carbs, proteins, and fats, as well as the concepts of glycemic index and glycemic load.

CHAPTER THREE

Building a Healthy Plate, Using the Plate Method, and Including a Variety of Foods are covered in Chapter 3.

The idea of a healthy plate develops as a cornerstone of informed eating in the context of managing diabetes. The skill of designing a plate that not only helps you achieve your blood sugar objectives but also encourages a wide variety of delicious nutrients is covered in Chapter 3. We provide tips for coordinating your meals and enjoying a range of healthy foods, from portion management to the creative plate technique.

The Magic of Moderation: Portion Control

Portion management orchestrates the symphony of nutrients on your plate, just like an expert conductor might. This chapter explains the power of moderation and the impact that serving size may have on your health. a significant effect on blood glucose levels. With the aid of useful tips and visual signals, you'll be able to confidently manage portion sizes, turning eating into an act of balanced mindfulness.

A Visual Symphony Using the Plate Method

Consider your plate as a painting, with each segment representing a balanced nutritional stroke. You can use the plate approach, a visual framework, to allocate quantities of vegetables, meats, and carbs. This chapter reveals the grace of this strategy, which makes meal preparation easier while fostering stable blood sugar levels and general wellbeing.

Adopting Cultural Diversity

Diversity becomes a prized advantage on your diabetes journey in a world full of many tastes, textures, and cultures. This chapter encourages you to accept a variety of cuisines as a way to appreciate the palette of possibilities. colorful vegetables You'll learn how to arrange your food on your plate with colors that reflect life and health, using lean meats and complete grains.

The Dance of Nutrients and Fiber

Because it helps maintain stable blood sugar levels, satiety, and gut health, fiber emerges as a dependable partner in the control of diabetes. This chapter clarifies the function of fiber-rich foods in your diet so you can make decisions that will satisfy both your physical and mental needs.

Making artistic meals

By fully committing to this chapter, you will develop the skill of preparing artistic meals. You'll plan meals that embody balance, diversity, and healthfulness if you use portion management and the plate method as your compass. Your plate's canvas changes into a wellness palette, where each option is a decision. demonstrates your dedication to self-care and diabetes management.

Beyond the Plate: A Healthful Way of Life

You go one step closer to mastering the complex dance of assembling a nutritious plate with every page you flip. You'll learn that this chapter is more than just about meals as you learn how to manage portions, embrace the plate approach, and taste a variety of foods. Instead, it's a first step towards a holistic lifestyle in which conscious eating becomes second nature. Your commitment to taking care of your body, mind, and diabetes journey will be reflected on your plate.

CHAPTER FOUR

Smart Food Choices: Best Sources of Carbohydrates for Blood Sugar Stability; Lean Proteins for Sustained Energy; Heart-Healthy Fats Chapter 4

The decisions you make when choosing meals build the fundamental foundation of your wellbeing in the mosaic of diabetic nutrition. Chapter 4 walks you through the maze of carbs, proteins, and fats as it unravels the tapestry of wise dietary selections. This chapter is a compass pointing you in the direction of meals that boost your vitality. It covers everything from stable blood sugar to prolonged energy and heart health.

Carbohydrates: The Smart Choice

In your body, carbohydrates act as keys to release energy. But not all keys are made equal. This chapter gives you the knowledge to recognize the best sources of carbohydrates: ones that release energy gradually, reducing blood sugar spikes, and ones that promote weight loss. crashes. You'll find the jewels that fuel your body without upsetting its equilibrium, such as nutritious grains and fiber-rich veggies.

Your allies for energy: lean proteins

The dependable building blocks of nourishment, proteins, provide more than simply sustenance for muscles. Lean proteins become your energy buddies, supplying your body with fuel while putting as little stress as possible on your blood sugar levels. This chapter clarifies protein-rich choices that support your objectives for managing your diabetes and offers guidance on how to skillfully incorporate them into your meals.

Healthy Fats for the Heart: Fueling Vitality

Fats, which are sometimes misinterpreted, are crucial for a balanced diet. The idea of heart-healthy fats is emphasized in this chapter, which also explains how they contribute to cardiovascular health. Avocado, almonds, and fatty fish are just a few of the alternatives you have to discover how to include these fats in your diet. taking care of both your physical and emotional needs.

The Influence of Food Pairing

Discover the power of food matching as you read this chapter to learn how to make proteins, carbs, and fats dance harmoniously together. You'll discover how to prepare balanced meals that maintain energy levels throughout the day while also balancing blood sugar. Your dining room table becomes a painting of food and vigor when you are aware of this.

'Nutritional Armory'

When you finish Chapter 4, you'll have a nutritious toolkit—a collection of wise food selections that fit in well with your lifestyle. With a solid grasp of the best types of carbs, lean proteins, and heart-healthy fats, you can create meals that support your fitness goals. Your plate serves as a palette. Every decision you make paints a masterpiece of diabetes control and vibrant life on the canvas of wellbeing.

CHAPTER FIVE

Chapter 5: Meal Preparation and Planning Includes Weekly Meal Planning advice and quick and simple diabetic-Friendly recipes.

The notes of meal planning and preparation carry weight in the symphony of diabetes control. The art of staging your meals with elegance is revealed in Chapter 5, which also includes a collection of fast and simple diabetic-friendly recipes that balance convenience and nutrition with weekly meal planning advice that transcends the routine.

Weekly Meal Preparation: A Guide to Success

Meal planning is more than just a habit; it's a guide for overcoming diabetes. This chapter reveals the power of intentionally planning your week, from developing menus to making grocery lists. You'll learn how forethought transforms meals into a fluid ballet of nourishment as you get into the rhythm of weekly meal planning.

Ingredients for Your Color Scheme

The story of sustenance and taste that each component tells brings to life the canvas of meal preparation. The elements that take center stage in your culinary symphony are honored in this chapter. You'll discover the world of options that add brightness to your meals while staying on your diabetic-friendly path, from fresh vegetables to cupboard staples.

Recipes that are quick and simple: Flavor in a Snap

Recipes that combine convenience and flavor are required by life's pace. This chapter provides a wealth of fast and simple diabetic-friendly meals that satisfy your cravings for food without sacrificing your health objectives. You'll find yourself whipping up delicious dinners in a matter of minutes, from colorful salads to one-pan marvels, leaving plenty of time for the pleasures of life outside the kitchen.

Nutrition and Simplicity in Balance

You'll learn how to balance nutrition and simplicity as you go through this chapter. The potential to create menus that satisfy your blood sugar requirements while embracing a variety of flavors arises through weekly meal planning. The recipes offered are not only culinary works of art; rather, they are an invitation to make cooking a pleasurable and self-indulgent activity.

You'll discover the lyrical core of meal preparation and planning with each page you turn. You'll set off on a culinary adventure that transcends subsistence, becoming a reflection of your dedication to health and vitality. You'll be armed with weekly meal planning ideas and a selection of quick and simple diabetic-friendly recipes. Your kitchen becomes a haven for inspiration and well-being.

CHAPTER FIVE

Managing Cravings and Emotional Eating is covered in Chapter 6's section on snacking strategies.

The time in between meals is crucial to the overall picture of managing diabetes. In Chapter 6, the topic of snacking tactics is covered in detail, showing how making wise decisions during these periods may help you achieve your blood sugar targets. This chapter walks readers over the fine line between nourishing themselves and indulging themselves, from carefully chosen snack selections to dealing with cravings and emotional eating.

Food for Thought: Nourishment in Bites

Snacking is a chance for conscious nourishment, not merely a means of satisfying hunger. This chapter reveals a plethora of clever snack alternatives that not only satisfy your palate but also support your goals for managing your diabetes. You'll enjoy everything from protein-packed nibbles to fiber-rich morsels.

Blood Sugar Balance with Snacks

When you use snacking to maintain a healthy blood sugar level, it becomes an artistic endeavor. This chapter gives you tips on how to strategically include snacks into your day to avoid energy slumps and maintain stable blood sugar levels. You'll discover that snacks are essential parts of your diabetes control symphony, with each note adding to the melody of the whole.

Decoding the Melody Cravings

Even the strictest regimens can be tested by cravings—those complex notes that dance within your palette. This chapter explores the psychology of cravings, identifies their causes, and offers strategies for controlling them. With knowledge, you'll be better equipped to handle urges and make decisions that align with your health goals.

Blood Sugar Balance with Snacks

When you use snacking to maintain a healthy blood sugar level, it becomes an artistic endeavor. This chapter gives you tips on how to strategically include snacks into your day to avoid energy slumps and maintain stable blood sugar levels. You'll discover that snacks are essential parts of your diabetes control symphony, with each note adding to the melody of the whole.

Decoding the Melody Cravings

Even the strictest regimens can be tested by cravings—those complex notes that dance within your palette. This chapter explores the psychology of cravings, identifies their causes, and offers strategies for controlling them. With knowledge, you'll be better equipped to handle urges and make decisions that align with your health goals.

CHAPTER SEVEN

Chapter 7: Recipes for Success Includes breakfast suggestions, lunch, and dinner recipes, plus options for snacks and desserts.

Chapter 7 stands out as a gold mine of carefully crafted recipes in the culinary voyage of managing diabetes. This chapter reveals a culinary repertoire that couples flavor with blood sugar harmony, starting with the first rays of morning and continuing with the magnificent spreads of lunch and dinner, as well as the delightful moments of snacks and desserts.

Breakfast Suggestions to Energize Your Day

Your meal transforms into a blank canvas for invigorating the hours ahead as dawn arrives. This chapter reveals a variety of breakfast concepts that give you morning energy. You'll go on a gastronomic adventure that lays the stage for stable blood sugar and protein levels, starting with substantial oatmeal varieties and protein-packed smoothies.

Recipes for lunch and dinner that are nourishing delights

Your gastronomic symphony's crescendos occur at lunch and dinner. A variety of meals that blend nutrition and flavor are introduced in this chapter. You'll learn how to create dishes that not only delight your palate but also support your goals for managing your diabetes, from colorful salads to healthy stir-fries.

Options for Snacks and Desserts: Indulgence with Intention

Snacks and sweets, which are sometimes associated with gluttony, turn into enjoyable occasions. This chapter offers a variety of snack choices that perfectly mix flavor and blood sugar stability. You'll also examine dessert concoctions that make sweetness a harmonic aspect of your diabetic journey.

Making Culinary Magic from the Kitchen to the Table

You'll go to the core of creating culinary magic with each dish provided. Your kitchen becomes your retreat as nutritious works of art are created through the alchemy of ingredients. You'll enjoy the satisfaction of cooking with intention as each dish connects with your health ambitions, from breakfast to dessert.

Beyond the Plate: A Legacy in Culinary Arts

You'll come to understand that these dishes are more than simply gourmet masterpieces as you progress through this chapter. They are also a legacy you leave behind. They demonstrate your dedication to good health, overall wellbeing, and effective diabetes treatment. You will be creating a culinary legacy with every mouthful you appreciate and every meal you savor that speaks of resiliency, balance, and the lovely nexus between flavor and health.

Conclusion
Final Thoughts: Taking Control of Your Diabetes Journey

You are about to embark on a magnificent adventure that will combine your knowledge of diabetes with the skill of properly fueling your body and promoting your wellbeing as we draw the curtain on this book. The chapters you've read are more than just words; they're beacons of empowerment and knowledge that point you in the direction of taking control of your diabetes journey.

This trip has demonstrated your tenacity, dedication, and unyielding spirit. With knowledge about diabetic nutrition, meal planning, wise food selections, and the ability to create culinary pleasures, you have a toolbox at your disposal that enables you to approach each day with confidence and purpose.

You've mastered the art of balancing the presence of carbs, proteins, and fats on your plate by learning to dance with them. You've delved deeply into food preparation and planning, turning your kitchen into a haven of creativity and good health. The once-casual activity of snacking has transformed into a deliberate routine that benefits both body and mind.

You've worked culinary magic by combining components to create healthful compositions that please the senses and respect blood sugar targets. Every food, from breakfast to dessert, embodies your passion for health and is evidence of how determined you are to master diabetes control.

Please keep in mind that you are in control of your diabetes journey as you read these pages. With information, being fed by purpose, and being directed by the knowledge acquired, You confidently go into a life that is balanced, energetic, and in line with your goals.

You are on a path of empowerment as you take control of your health. You create the melodies of your life as the conductor of this symphony, fusing the harmony of vitality with the notes of diabetes control. You confirm with each action, decision, and meal that you are not simply managing your diabetes but also leading a strong, fulfilling life.

So, my friend, go on this trip knowing that you are not traveling alone. The light of knowledge, the wisdom of a healthy diet, and the strength of taking initiative all shine on the route you travel. Your battle with diabetes is not a burden; it's a chance to live resiliently, to appreciate each moment, and to compose a health symphony that resounds with power and elegance.